THE HEALING POWERS OF
GARLIC

Nature's Ancient Medicine
in Modern, Deodorized Form

by
Morton Walker, D.P.M.

NEW WAY OF LIFE, INC.
1845 Summer Street
Stamford, Connecticut 06905

A LIFE ENHANCEMENT BOOK

Published by NEW WAY OF LIFE, Inc.
1845 Summer Street
Stamford, Connecticut 06905 U.S.A.
(203) 322-1551 or (203) 323-2808
Distributed in Canada by Abramson Publishing, Ltd.
Distributed in Great Britain by Alphavite Publications Ltd.

Copyright • 1988 by Morton Walker, D.P.M.

ISBN Number 0-945498-00-4

Library of Congress Catalog Card Number 88-90582

Disclaimer

This book has been written and published strictly for informational purposes, and in no way should it be used as a substitute for advice from your own physician, nutritional counselor, or other health care professional.

You should not consider educational material found here to replace consultation with a medical practitioner. However, almost all the facts have come from medical files, scientific publications, and personal interviews with informed physicians and their patients who have suffered from low levels of wellness, subclinical illness, or outright disease. For centuries, people have sought relief of discomforts by employing raw clove garlic. Then they turned to processed and refined garlic, aged garlic extract, and, more recently, forms of deodorized or odor-modified garlic.

Many have discovered that processed, deodorized garlic is useful for soothing or healing purposes. Eager to share this knowledge, they are using the author and publisher as their means for such sharing with others. True Case histories are included along with direct quotes from physicians who have recorded them. All the health care professionals mentioned are in practice and may be contracted for more information. However, the names of most patients have been changed to protect their identities.

Table of Contents

The Healing/Curing Powers of Garlic

What is the difference between disease and illness? Disease is a pathological entity, frequently defined by signs of a lesion such as an ulcer, tumor, or abscess. The lesion may possess characteristics which clearly demarcate the disease. Or, the disease may offer clues in the form of specific symptoms which can be observed, leading to an exact differential diagnosis. A disease theoretically has a cure, which has been developed through the use of the scientific method.

Illness, on the other hand, is the wholistic perception by a patient of his or her symptoms, such as pain, nausea, dizziness, etc. An illness may not have a specific cure but can sufficiently heal by itself or from the intervention of an outside agent which soothes symptoms or allows the patient comfort.

Through its development of medical science, mankind searches perpetually for the universal healing/curing agent. New Age nostrums, Eastern health practices, folklore of foreign cultures, allopathic experimentations, homeopathic discoveries, herbal remedies, and other forms of esoterica are constantly being explored for products and techniques of treatment for healing and/or cure. Many patients visit physicians expecting to be healed, while physicians are busy examining, testing, and diagnosing in preparation to cure. This dichotomy—the patient's desire to be healed, the doctor's intention to cure—seemingly comes together in one ancient herbal medicine: garlic.

Today, the much loved stinking rose, garlic, scientifically known as *Allium sativum*, is packaged in new and convenient dress—without the smell. Wonder workings of modern science bring us an aged, deodorized garlic extract with its enhanced ability to heal/cure a variety of ills.

Thanks to nutritional research, scientific testing, new methods of processing, and high technology packaging, the offense to one's nose which was manifested by chopped, sliced, ground, mashed, or grated garlic has been eliminated. Now you may acquire the beneficial ingredients in garlic and make them a part of your food supply without introducing garlic's characteristic odor to others in your immediate vicinity. This small book describes the healing/curing powers of aged, odor-modified extract of garlic, nature's ancient herbal medicine as a modern, processed, packaged remedy.

The Healing Properties of Garlic in Recorded History

In Sanskrit, the earliest known written language, the healing/curing properties of garlic were first recorded on parchment text pages about 5,000 years ago.

Two thousand years later, Chinese scholars praised this potent member of the lily family, asserting that it contained the medicinal qualities to cure and prevent virtually any illness.

Thus, garlic has been known as a food and medicine for many thousands of years. The children of Israel complained on their long journey from Egypt that there was no garlic and onion, both being members of the plant family of alliums (which also includes leeks and shallots.) The book of NUMBERS 11:5 reads:

We remember the fish, which we did eat in Egypt freely; the cucumbers, and the melons, and the leeks, and the onions, and the garlic.

The ancient pyramid builders made raw garlic a part of their food ration. They said that it gave them stamina. (Today, the stamina-producing qualities of garlic have been proven in animal laboratories and will be reported to you in the next section.) According to the Talmud, garlic is useful to stop hunger pangs, brighten the face, improve the circulation, keep the body warm, kill parasites, and give strength to laborers.

According to the historian, Herodotus of Greece, Egyptian laborers building the great pyramid of Cheops for King Herod went on strike and refused to work until their meals included sufficient garlic to maintain their health, strength, and stamina. The King spent the equivalent of two million American dollars purchasing garlic from farmers near and far to feed his workers.

Warriors and adventurers such as the Phoenicians, and later the Vikings, packed garlic in their sea chests when they began their lengthy voyages. For them, the herb was their healer of ills and a giver of strength.

In 400 B.C., both Hippocrates, the "father of medicine," and

Pliny the Elder, his disciple, a naturalist and physician, wrote of the powerful therapeutic properties displayed by this herb. Pliny listed over sixty diseases that could be treated effectively with garlic. He said, "Garlic has such a powerful smell that it drives away serpents and scorpions." (We know that woodsmen and hikers nowadays do employ it topically and internally to repel mosquitoes and tiny black flies.) Pliny also affirmed that it cures respiratory and tubercular ailments.

In the first century A.D., garlic was part of the prescribed diet for the Roman Legions.

The Irish, Danish, and Russians have used garlic for centuries (and still do) for coughs and colds. In Ireland, it is a primary household remedy for chronic bronchitis.

In World War I the British Army doctors controlled wound infections by topical applications of sliced raw clove garlic.

Albert Schweitzer and the Bircher-Benner Clinic in Europe applied garlic as a cure for everything from intestinal disorders and stomach problems to hypertension, senility, and impotence.

Indeed, throughout recorded history, you will find continual references to the miraculous benefits attributed to eating garlic. It appears to have been the accepted panacea for just about every ailment known to mankind.

As people became more civilized, however, they started to be concerned about offending others. In our modern world, of course, many don't wish to jeopardize social relationships by eating raw garlic before going out in public. If garlic then, is able to accomplish all of its purported benefits, how can one have the best of it without disclosing the worst of it?

The answer to the garlic odor dilemma was discovered in Japan about thirty years ago. It was found in a whole clove garlic extract that retains all of the natural beneficial qualities of raw garlic without any residual odor. Aged garlic extract which has been odor-modified is now available at a few supermarkets, some pharmacies, most mail order nutritional outlets, and all health food stores around the world.

This unique product—aged and deodorized garlic liquid, tablets, or capsules—along with its malodorous parent has become the subject of an increasing number of research projects and published scientific papers. Unlike raw clove garlic, however, the extract of odor-modified garlic has *not* been known to cause irritation to the intestinal tract or stomach. So people everywhere now have a natural weapon against disease and sub-clinical illness without side effects from the treatment.

Specifically, what can garlic do for you? How might it be your own healer/cure for what ails you? Information on the following pages contains researched facts that might surprise you and even give you hope of healing where none existed before. But remember, as important as aged, deodorized garlic extract may be, healing and curativeness, good health, longevity, and an improved quality of life also require a proper diet, probably nutritional supplementation, regularly scheduled exercise, rest and relaxation, occasional supervision by a physician, and other wholistic methods of self-maintenance. Garlic usage can be an adjunctive supplement to these optimal health techniques.

Animal Tests for Garlic's Effects on Stamina, Resistance to Fatique, and Recovery

At the Central Research Laboratories in Hiroshima, Japan, the antistress effects of odor-modified, aged garlic extract were tested on laboratory animals. I visited those laboratories and observed the testing taking place. A variety of stringent physical examinations were performed on the animals before and after garlic was administered and before and after tests were con-ducted.

The animals were subjected to stress. For example, ten control mice and ten mice given garlic were stressed by placing them on a reciprocating shaker apparatus at 129 excursions per minute for four hours. Physiological tests were performed before stress, immediately after, and 30 minutes after exposure to the oscilla-tion stimulus.

Measurements were then taken of the mice's rectal tempera-ture with an ordinary rectal thermometer.

Measurements were made on the mouse spring balance test. In this test, a mouse is placed on a small metal net which con-nects to a spring balance, and then it is pulled backwards by the

In this test, a mouse is placed on a small metal net which connects to a spring balance, and then it is pulled backwards by the tail. The reading at which the mouse fails to hold onto the net is automatically recorded on a kymograph.

Measurements were made on the mouse sliding angle test. In this test, a motor-driven plastic plate is inclined at a speed of 103 degrees per minute from horizontal. The critical angle at which the mouse falls is taken as the sliding angle score.

Measurements were made on the mouse rotating rod test. In this test, a plastic rod 3.2 cm in diameter is rotated at a speed of 12 rotations per minute (rpm). Mice which fell off the rod in three minutes were taken to be exhibiting incoordination; only those mice which stayed on the rotating rod for more than five minutes in two successive trials were given a positive score.

Measurements were made on the mouse exploratory movement test. In this test, a box with three compartments—two outer transparent compartments connected to a darkened middle one by two round openings—measures three kinds of exploratory movements and one spontaneous movement of mice.

Measurements were made on the mouse motor activity test. The number of times that a mouse climbed into the second hole in the exploratory movement apparatus were averaged.

Measurements were also made of mice under cold stress. The animals were kept in a cold room at 4 degrees centigrade for three weeks with free access to food and water. The animals' fatigue was recorded by noting their rectal temperature, body weight, food consumption, and water consumption.

It was found that the mice given garlic showed signs of remarkably less fatigue, greater stamina, and faster recovery than the controls when they were checked for rectal temperature, spring balance ability, sliding angle ability, rotating rod ability, motor activity, and exploratory movement following stress.

In addition, garlic was compared to other nutrients or drugs administered to the mice for its effects on recovery and on prevention against loss of stamina and early onset of fatigue. Garlic far surpassed the recovery and preventive effects of caffeine, glucose, ginseng, and six other food and drug items commonly used to restore energy, produce alertness, give vigor, or furnish endurance. *Allium sativum* offered the animals greater vitality and more power to endure against stress.

In summary, laboratory tests on animals have been conclusive in proving the general recovery benefits, antifatigue factors, and stamina-maintaining powers of aged, deodorized garlic extract. The question is, might odor-modified garlic's positive effects in animals be translated to similar effects on humans?

Aged, Dedorized Garlic Extract as the Universal Human Healer

Fifty-two-year-old Allen Broudy, an electrical engineer from Lincoln, Nebraska, felt constant bone and joint pain. He was the victim of rheumatoid arthritis, among other health troubles. Every day for over ten years Broudy swallowed six 600-milligram (mg) buffered aspirin of a recognizable physician-prescribed brand [a triple-ingredient anti-inflammatory pain-killing drug]. His belief was that taking two of these pills as he did, three times a day, allowed him to cope with the arthritic pain.

"I had been an athletic person much of my working life, but for the past decade soreness of the joints, fatigue, and an inability to get physically and mentally started in the morning kept me from performing on the tennis court or in other sports. Although there were possible side effects with taking the pain-killer, I swallowed it anyway in order to go without rheumatic joint pain. When the drug's effect wore off, however, I worried about being in bad shape between doses. So, I looked for various natural remedies to assist me, not only with the joint pain but with several other health problems, too," Mr. Broudy said.

"I had high blood pressure, was prone to depression, felt a need to push myself beyond what my bodily functions were able to do, experienced mental confusion, constantly had aching shoulders and arms, and my sore knees felt like they were weighted down with lead. I could hardly lift my legs to walk. The skin on my feet was blistering and breaking all the time. My feet itched with athlete's foot. Also I had general muscle pain, drained energies, frequent insomnia, gastrointestinal distress, and a few different sexual troubles such as impotence," added Broudy.

"Furthermore, for years I required a bulk-forming laxative [another popular brand] for chronic constipation. In short, two months ago I was a mess. But now that's all changed," he said. "In my local health food store, I read literature about deodorzied garlic. The magazine article—in fact, written by you, Dr. Walker—described ordinary whole clove garlic grown in purified, well-nourished soil in Japan. The Japanese technicians pick the cloves when they are ripe and age them in huge vats. Then the garlic is laboratory-tested, factory-processed, made into liquid, powder, capsules, and tablets, and sold around the world as aged garlic extract. Such processing and packaging causes the garlic to permanently lose its odor.

"It happens that my mother was a great exponent of using raw clove garlic as an herbal remedy. She gave it to me when I was a child. As an adult, I didn't eat garlic anymore, because of the breath odor it left," Broudy said. "According to what I read, many medicinal properties ascribed to the aged, deodorized garlic would directly benefit me. So I bought a supply and tried it."

He explained the results. "I took nine capusles filled with deodorized garlic powder every day, three after each meal. In one week I saw improvements in myself. First, my feet stopped itching and the athlete's foot blebs disappeared. The next week I noticed that no more muscle joint soreness came on between my doses of prescription aspirin," Broudy said. "The drug's pain-killing effects either lasted longer or I didn't need the arthritis pain-killer anymore. It wasn't until the third week that I began experimenting with reducing my pain pill dosage. It became less and less. Now I don't take aspirin or any other type of drug to relieve arthritis symptoms. My joint inflammation and pain are simply gone. Muscles in my shoulders, arms, and knees have stopped feeling sore, as well.

"There's no more extreme fatigue for me either," said the man. "In all categories my body appears to be functioning better. Insomnia doesn't keep me awake any longer. In the second week of taking deodorized garlic, my blood pressure went to normal and has remained there. My mind is alert all the time now so that confusion doesn't befuddle me," he said.

"I didn't mention that I had allergies to some foods, certain food additives, cigarette smoke, and miscellaneous items. For the past couple of months, since I am supplmenting with deodorized, aged garlic extract, I have no more allergic reactions such as emotional depression, headache, stomach upset, skin rash, and other common discomforts," said the electrical engineer. "They just don't come on anymore, even if I'm intimately exposed to my personal powerful allergens. The garlic has overcome them.

"When I also began taking the newly developed combination capsules of aged garlic extract with added ginseng powder, my sexual problems went away," affirmed Broudy. "Ejaculate reappeared and impotence was cured. My wife and I have been enjoing a renewal of our sex lives again." (At this point in the interview, Mrs. Helen Broudy nodded enthusiastically.)

Four weeks ago I added deodorized liquid garlic to my regimen, and constipation is no longer my problem either. I ran out of stool-forming laxative a week after beginning the liquid, but my bowel movements have been so steady and well-formed that taking laxatives aren't part of my daily routine anymore. Deodorized garlic is a fine bowel stimulator. It seems to have settled down my lower colon and balanced the rest of my gastrointestinal tract," Broudy declared. "For this purpose alone—ridding myself of body wastes in comfort every day—I would recommend taking daily doses of deodorized garlic. It acts on me as a natural diuretic too.

"I surely wouldn't want to be without this convenient, modern herbal medicine—aged, deodorized garlic extract. It acted as a cure for my many disease conditions. How did garlic work? I don't know for sure, but I believe it helped my body heal itself. Now I'm rid of muscle soreness, high blood pressure, sex trouble, athlete's foot, constipation, allergy symptoms, arthritis, insomnia, depression, mental confusion, fatigue, and probably other troubles of which I was less aware," said Allen Broudy. "In my opinion, aged garlic extract is among the best all-purpose food supplements available in any health food store. I wouldn't be without it."

Thus, confirming ancient wisdom relating to raw clove garlic from centuries past, garlic that is aged, processed, deodorized, and packaged in modern wrappings often is judged positively and with favor by many uncomfortable people who suffer from various symptoms. They see improvements in their health. Using nonscientific terms but making valid observations, they advocate this herbal medication to improve the quality of life by health enhancement. Like Allen Broudy, troubled persons may have discomforts from body breakdown that are not readily measurable. To them it matters not why a remedy gives relief. These patients merely want their discomforts to go away. The healing/curative properties of deodorized garlic therefore become meaningful for the well-being of anyone with physical, mental, or emotional discomforts.

Healing Ingredients in Garlic

What is there in garlic that gives it healing/curative properties or makes it useful against disruption of the immune system, cancer, cardiovascular disorders, arthritis, chronic infections, and other autoimmune and degenerative diseases? The nutritional content of the average-size clove of garlic has been determined by the United States Department of Agriculture. One clove provides 7 calories of energy; 0.31 gms of protein; 0.01 gms of carbohydrate; 1.4 mg of calcium; 10 mg of phosphorus; 0.07 mg of iron; 0.9 mg of sodium; 26 mg of potassium; 0.01 mg of thiamin (vitamin B-1); 0.004 mg (i.e. 4 mcg) of riboflavin (vitamin B-2); 0.02 mg of niacin (vitamin B-3); and 0.75 mg of ascorbic acid (vitamin C).

There are also seventy-five sulfur-containing compounds in garlic whose listing might possibly be of interest to biochemists, nutritionists, physiologists, chemists, physicians, or other physical scientists but not necessarily to the average reader. To give just a few of them, they include: allicin, diallysulfide, cysteic acid, methionine, alliin, and the crystalline isolates from *Allium sativum* such as S-methyl cysteine and cycloalliin.

This garlic herb also contains specific nutritive value by its makeup of seventeen amino acids, including the eight essential ones. The human body requires twenty amino acids to build pro-

tein, but half of these can be synthesized within the body. The
ones labeled "essential" must be derived from food sources such
as garlic. (Those listed here with a single asterisk [*] beside them
are the essential ones. The two amino acids listed here with double asterisks [**] are considered semi-essential.) The amino acids
contained in garlic are:

*lysine	*phenylalanine	alanine
*valine	*leucine	proline
*methionine	*threonine	aspartic acid
*isoleucine	**histidine	serine
*tryptophan	**arginine	glutamine
cysteine	glycine	

Even more than these nutritional advantages, refined or raw
garlic has in it certain other identifiable therapeutic factors
which come from the herb's nutrient content. Garlic's important
health enhancement factors have been experienced by patients
of progressive clinicians who practice wholistic medicine using
nutrition in preference to drugs as therapeutic agents. Such physicians have reported the beneficial effects of garlic by publishing scientific papers about garlic's therapeusis in their wholistic
medical journals, newsletters and magazines. They have also
reported personal experiences from the lecture platform when
furthering the knowledge of their colleagues.

Health Enchancement Factors in Raw or Refined Garlic

a. *Radiation antidote factor* derives from a mitogenetic alex-
ipharmic (presevative against poison) that is part of the herb's
synergistic combination of constituents. Garlic's antidote coun-
teracts radiation toxicity. It stimulates cellular detoxification,
organelle growth, and cellular membrane restoration, and brings
about subsequent general rejuvenation of body functions.

b. *Antihemolytic factor* is responsible for the herb's beneficial
effect on anemia, leukemia, and other blood dyscrasias.

c. *Antiarthritic factor* reduces joint inflammation and swelling
by its tendency to proliferate fibrotic growth among ligaments
and other connective tissues. Garlic has become an adjunctive
nutrient presecribed by physicians with an interest in the mus-

culoskeletal system who apply proliferative therapy for the elimination of chronic joint pain. Proliferative therapy involves the injection of a derivative of pharmaceutical grade cod liver oil, called sodium morrhuate, which acts as an irritant to cause the body to send healing cells (fibroblasts) to bring about a natural repair in the injected ligamentous attachments of the affected joints.

d. *Sugar metabolism factor* makes this lily-bulb derivative useful for treating both diabetes and hypoglycemia, as well as other irregularities of insulin metabolism.

e. *Chelation factor* comes from vast quantities of *selenium and germanium* packed into the bulb. The garlic plant absorbs these two nutritionally necessary minerals from the soil exceedingly well. This high absorption phenomenon occurs because selenium, in particular, has a chemical structure distinctly similar to sulfur. And sulfur attracts the molecules in garlic, perhaps through an herbal plant chelation (bonding) process. Consequently, among practically all plants, garlic contains the highest level of the antioxidant selenium with its chelation-like substitution effect on impurities within the blood vessels and body cells.

f. *Antiheavy metal factor* seemingly works by chelation within the blood stream to neutralize heavy metal toxicity. Indeed, organically grown garlic is the most effective form of oral chelation therapy known to be available.

g. *Antioxidant factor* reduces lipid peroxides and other free radical end-products (see the next subsection for a fuller explanation).

h. *Allithiamine factor* forms by the action of vitamin B-1 (thiamine) on the sulfur-containing compound alliin.

I. *Antibiotic factor* gets produced by the action of the enzyme alliinase on alliin. This factor increases the immune system's resistance against bacterial infection. In the article "The Antimicrobial Activity of Garlic and Onion Extract," (see *Pharmazie*, 38:747-748, 1983), E. Elnima and coworkers reported that garlic reduces the infectious effect of *Staphylococcus* (staph infection), *Streptococcus* (strep infection), *Vibrio* cholerae (cholera), *Corynebacterium* diphtheriae (diphtheria), *Rickettsia* rickettsii (typhus), and *Shigella* enteritides (bacillary dysentery).

It's well known among travelers in Mexico, India, and other places where the purity of drinking water remains uncertain that aged garlic extract will protect you against acute infection of the bowel, otherwise known as "bush-to-bush" disease. Eric Block, Ph.D., Professor of Chemistry at the State University of New York at Albany, in "The Chemistry of Garlic and Onions" (*Scientific American*, 252: 114-119, 1985) stated, "Laboratory investigations show that garlic juice diluted to one part in 125,000 inhibits the growth of bacteria."

In the article, "Garlic in Cryptococcal Meningitis, a Preliminary Report of 21 Cases" (*Chinese Medical Journal*, 93:123-126, 1980), the editors reported that in a major Chinese hospital treatment with garlic was used effectively against cryptococcal meningitis, which is one of the AIDS (autoimmune deficiency syndrome) infections. The article editors indicated that natural garlic extract can cross the blood-brain barrier and enter into brain tissue, unlike most synthetic drugs which cannot.

j. *Antifungal factor* in the herb is exhibited both by experiments in the body and in the laboratory. Garlic has demonstrated its ability as a fungicidal agent to be more potent than many commercial antifungal drugs, including the generic antifungal antibiotic drug, nystatin, for The Yeast Syndrome (candidiasis). Ingested *Allium sativum* combats *Candida albicans*, the causative fungus of The Yeast Syndrome, by actually reversing its growth. These last two statements are paraphrased from the article by Drs. F. Barone and M. Tansey, "Isolation, Purification, Synthesis, and Kinetic Activity of the Anticandidal Component of *Allium sativum*, and a Hypothesis for Its Mode of Action" (*Mycologia* 69: 793-825, 1977). Garlic also is fungicidal against the organisms: *Epidermophyton*, *Trichophyton*, and *Microsporum*.

k. *Antiparasitic factor* works against intestinal parasites such as giardia and cryptosporidia. The ancient herbal remedy has been used with success throughout human history for intestinal worms and other parasites of the gastrointestinal tract.

l. *Anti-inflammatory factor* comes directly from allicin, an unstable substance changing into diallyl sulfide and diallyl disulfide at room temperature within 20 hours after the garlic blub has been crushed. As mentioned, allicin is one of garlic's many sulfur compounds which have therapeutic properties. While allicin is the primary substance which gives garlic its unpleasant odor, there are 19 other known constituents which produce garlic odor as well. Pharmacologist Willis R. Brewer, Ph.D., Dean and Professor Emeritus, College of Pharmacy, University of Arizona, says, "Allicin is not solely responsible for garlic odor. Some processors of garlic products use heat to kill enzymes in order to reduce garlic odor. Once enzymes are destroyed, there is little conversion of alliin to allicin and resulting beneficial compounds."

m. *Antihypertensive factor* in garlic is recognized by the Japanese Food and Drug Administration. Prescribing aged garlic extract is practically standard treatment among Japanese physicians for lowering their patients' elevated blood pressures.

n. *Antihypercholesteremic factor* decreases elevated blood cholesterol, increases the blood's protective lipid called HDL, and normalizes a recipient's blood fat profile.

o. *Anticoagulant factor* comes from ajoene, a compound in garlic that is believed by Dr. Eric Block to be efficacious in preventing blood platelets from sticking to, and thereby clogging, arterial walls. It also inhibits clumping of lymphocytes (one of the forms of white blood cells).

p. *Anticlotting factor* (adjunctive to ajoene) arises from the presence of methyltrisulfide (MATS). Japanese researchers have identified MATS as one of the key sulfur compounds responsible for the prevention of blood clots, thrombi, or emboli when garlic is ingested.

q. *Artery-cleansing factor* has been known to be present in garlic since 86 A.D. when Greek physicians recorded this benefit from eating the stinking rose. There is a lessened incidence of arterial disease in cultures where garlic-eating is popular, such as Italy, China, and Spain.

r. *Anticancer factor* is readily recorded not only in the history of garlic use through the ages but also more recently in Western medical literature. (See the sections on laboratory and clinical investigations of garlic for cancer, pages 23-28).

s. *Antiviral factor* occurring from six percent of the dry weight of garlic being made up of the *bioflavonoids quercitin and cyanidin.* They have antiviral, anti-inflammatory, and anti-oxidant properties.

t. *Vitamin factor* includes elevated quantities of the *vitamins B-1 (thiamin), B-2 (riboflavin), B-3 (niacin), C (ascorbate), and A (carotene).*

u. *Mineral factor* contained in the clove (in addition to selenium and germanium) consist of *calcium, iron, and zinc.*

v. *Protein factor* is present in garlic. It takes the form of amino acids cysteine, glutamine, isoleucine, methionine and others. The particular ones mentioned here also behave as free radical quenchers (see below, factor x).

w. *Miscellaneous therapeutic factor* in garlic has virtues which have been attributed to the presence of diallysulfide, unstable sulfur in alkyl polysulfides, and to a chemically undefined group of substances designated as phytoncides. Russian scientists believe that these phytoncides are the mysterious elements that make garlic a therapeutic food.

Veterinarians, using the miscellaneous therapeutic factor as the sole rationale for administering raw garlic, fed the herb to a group of horses in France suffering from peripheral vasular diseases of the veins with associated thromboses. This therapeutic garlic regimen poved to be quite effective as a corrective treatment.

x. *Anti-free-radical factor,* a form of chelation therapy, derives from garlic's sulfur-containing chemicals. It turns out that these sulfur compounds are scavengers of harmful free radicals in food additives, cigarette smoke, alcoholic beverages, radiation, and many other sources.

The anti-free-radical factor in garlic quenches the energy of free radicals to stop their pathological process within the cells. Garlic contains anti-oxidant nutrients which assume the role of efficient free radical quenchers, as well.

Disease Production from Free Radical Pathology

The presence in your body of a harmful molecular state known as free radical pathology is the source of premature aging and degenerative disease, and is the common determining factor for so-called "dying a natural death." The ordinarily occurring triple phenomena of aging, disease, and death are not themselves prime movers in life's regression. Instead, they are the results of recurring and cumulative free radical pathology.

A free radical is any cellular molecule in your body possessing an odd number of electrons which makes the molecule electrochemically unbalanced. This unbalancing act of an electrically charged form of an element gives it great affinity for reacting with other elements. Free radicals, especially those of oxygen, have been implicated in causing the kinds of genetic change in cells that lead to cancer.

Our bodies are composed of multi-trillions of molecules having multiquadrillions (unimaginable numbers) of electrons all spinning in molecular orbits. When the spinning remains stable, your body tissues function normally. It's a law of nature that electrons prefer to occur in pairs and are stabilized in the molecule by spinning in opposite directions. The phenomenon has to do with the fundamental symmetry of space and time. Asymmetry produces free radical pathology.

Thus, for whatever reason, if a single electron is caused to be present, the molecule will usually become unstable and set up an electrochemically detectable imbalance from the electromagnetic field that the single unpaired electron creates. This electrochemically imbalanced molecule is called a free radical, and is capable of doing harm to the tiny chemical factories called "organelles" located within each of the approximately 80 trillion cells of the average human body.

All of us are undergoing free radical bombardment without and within our bodies all of the time. If you are assaulted sufficiently, cellular damage results, tissue breakdown occurs, illness sets in, and finally you experience the development of disease. As you will learn here, aged and deodorized extract of garlic helps you to offset the effects of being bombarded with free radicals outside and inside the body.

Free Radical "Fireplace Sparks"

A way to visualize free radicals is to compare them to sparks popping from a burning log in a fireplace on a wintery day. Stephen Levine, Ph.D., Director of Research of Nutri-Cology, Inc. of San Leandro, California draws this burning log analogy for understanding free radical production. Writing in the spring 1984 *Allergy Research Review,* Dr. Levine states:

The burning of the wood provides needed heat energy. We have a good protective screen so that sparks from the fire don't damage our clothes or furniture. The sparks are part of the fire that have strayed from the fireplace, for which we need the screen. Think of that screen as composed of our antioxidant defense systems [from nutrients which we consume in food or as food supplements]. Think of the sparks as free radicals, which are a normal consequence of cellular metabolism [using energy to function], and represent certain inefficiencies in the burning process. The free radicals are potentially damaging if our screen is old or damaged. The numerous parts of our antioxidant defense system must absorb the potentially damaging sparks (free radicals).

Free radical production increases when we become overwhelmed by environmental chemical exposures, emotional stress, infection, physical injury, sharp temperature changes, radiation, or other abusive biological/chemical alterations of the body's equilibrium. It's like throwing a fresh log on the fire; more sparks are created.

What tangible items can you point to as producers of free radical sparks? They consist of unhealthful actions people engage in daily such as drinking cola beverages, artificial flavorings, impure water, alcohol, or coffee; using rancid salad dressing, rancid cooking oil or artificial sweeteners; inhaling tobacco smoke, including the passive or residual smoke from somebody else; getting sunburned; standing before a working microwave oven, television set, or a computer's video display terminal; accumulat-

ing too much X-irradiation, cosmic radiation, or nuclear radiation; eatng food additives such as foaming agents, preservatives,
colorings, and other shelf-life extenders; and personal exposure
to many more endogenous metabolic processes (inside oneself)
or exogenous chemicals or drugs (from our surroundings).
Whether your body has the ability to deal with these free radical sparks is dependent on its resiliency to stress which, in turn,
is directly related to its antioxidant defense capabilities. This may
be measured and evaluated as the balance of electromagnetic
forces affecting an electron. The measurement of this oxidation-
reduction reaction within your body has a name: "redox potential." One way that ingesting aged, deodorized garlic protects us
against free radical pathology is that it reinforces redox potential
from inside the body by using the individual's own antioxidant
defense system.

If antioxidant nutrients such as those present in garlic fail to be
an integral part of your daily food consumption, early aging and
degenerative diseases are likely to be your destiny. Free radical
pathology resulting from bombarding molecules which possess
unpaired electrons could be the death of you.

How Garlic Protects Against Free Radicals

Tobacco (and marijuana) smoke contains high concentrations
of free radicals which certainly react with the respiratory tract.
Smoking also increases the number of macrophages, which are
PAC MAN-like protection cells produced by the immune system
and located in the millions of lung air sacs. These cells try to eat
the cigarette smoke condensate and the cigarette's associated
tobacco tars. But macrophages produce considerable oxygen
radicals during these activities, which may contribute to the lung
damage that almost all chronic smokers develop. Free radicals
from single-electron oxygen molecules are the most common
kind.

The toxic free radicals and other noxious substances in
tobacco smoke circulate throughout the body to bring on much
damage. They incite the development of many types of cancers,
accelerate occulsive atherosclerosis, cause peptic ulcers, and

injure the lungs sometimes beyond self-repair by the body's healing mechanisms.

To protect you, where does garlic fit into this picture? As was mentioned earlier, garlic contains a number of amino acids which are necessary for the formation of an enzymatic antidote for the free radical pathology created by inhaling tobacco smoke (and most other pollutants). The amino acids required to counteract free radicals are the same ones that make up the nutritional ingredients in garlic. The amino acids such as cysteine, glutamine, isoleucine, and methionine present in aged garlic extract are your protectors against or healers of free radical pathology.

Also, garlic is heavy in selenium, germanium, niacin, riboflavin, and other nutrients which are instrumental in the body's metabolic antidote reaction. If you had consumed your share of garlic cloves or aged garlic extract before coming in contact with a smoker, you could cope with his or her smoke's polluting stressors that are so unhealthy and such an annoyance as you dine.

The Power of Aged Garlic Extract in the Immune System

Taking aged garlic extract may help prevent health problems tied to an underfunctioning immunity. This concept was considered in a clinical study by a staff physician at the Akbar Clinic and Research Institute in Panama City, Florida. Tariq Abdullah, M.D. advises that his research has proved garlic protects the body against cancer by stimulating the immune system. In experiments with three groups of volunteer cancer patients, early in 1987, Dr. Abdullah and his research team consisting of Ahmed Elkadi, M.D. and Osama Kandil, M.D. discovered that aged deodorized garlic works with more potency for enhancing immunity than does raw clove garlic.

Dr. Abdullah fed one group of patients a small amount of raw garlic every day for three weeks. A second group took capsules containing cold-aged garlic extract. A third group—the patients acting as controls—took no garlic at all. Dr. Abdullah's researchers then tested blood samples from each group for the activity of white blood cells (leucocytes), which medical science has identified as the body's guardians (killer cells) against cancer. Leucocytes checked from group one, those who ate the raw garlic, killed 139 percent more cancer cells than those from group three, the controls who ate no garlic. Killer cells taken from the second group, which took the capsules of Kyolic™ cold aged garlic extract destroyed 159 percent more tumor cells than cells taken from the control group.

At the start of 1988, Dr. Abdullah and his team began experiments to uncover if aged garlic extract can help to stimulate the body's immune system to fight herpes and AIDS. "Garlic kills a broad spectrum of disease-carrying organisms—from viruses, to bacteria [microscopic plants] to protozoa [microscopic animals]," says Dr. Abdullah.

Why might garlic's components enhance your immunity? Robert C. Atkins, M.D. of New York City offers a logical reason. He affirms, "Garlic is an important nutritional food. The most reasonable explanation for its effectiveness [as a contributor of power to the immune system] is that it picks up toxic materials and transports them out of the body."

Aged, odor-modified garlic brings balance to the immune system: that semblage of different organs, tissues, and chemicals; much of which cannot be seen with the naked eye or even with a microscope. The immune system acts as a second brain in our bodies and was long unrecognized by medical scientists simply because it is not a single organ but a very complex system of interrelated cellular structures.

Ingesting the food factors in garlic is fundamental to maintaining a viable immune system. Recent scientific studies have demonstrated that immune system changes occurring in autoimmune diseases are exact copies of immune system changes that occur in malnutrition.

Subclinical Illness from Too Much Stress

For whatever stressful reason—suffering with the common cold, inadequate nourishment, too much smoking, a degenerative disease, physical injury, chemical pollution, or some other burden—your body will fail to function at high level wellness (peak performance) because of the stress. The immune system is put under pressure to fight off the burden. Your body will then offer up a low level of wellness or subclinical illness (feeling symptoms without manifesting obvious signs of disease) or quite apparent indications of health impairment. In that case, consuming aged, deodorized garlic will work toward restoring your immune system. This ancient remedy in modern dress tends to bring the body's organelles, cells, hormones, enzymes, and other tissues and fluids back to normalcy.

The body in its wisdom knows what to do in each instance of lowered immunity. Your job as a person potentially performing at low level wellness or subclinical illness is to give your immune system all the help it can get. This means that you need to put the best nutrition into this body so that the five million white blood cells being made each minute in your bone marrow for purposes of immunity are of the strongest caliber.

Garlic furnishes this kind of fine nutrition from the components it contains: thiamine, sulfur compounds, niacin, phosphorous, selenium, and more. Most of all, it contains the immune system supporting power of germanium.

Immunity Stimulation from Garlic's Germanium

Other than shelf fungus (*Trametes cinnabarina Fr.*) which contains from 800 to 2000 parts per million (ppm) of germanium, the highest quantity of this therapeutic mineral found in any plant is present in garlic. According to Kazuhiko Asai, Ph.D. (now deceased) of the Asai Germanium Research Institute, Tokyo, Japan, certain plant and animal proteins regarded as having medicinal qualities and conducive to good health are ones with the greatest concentrations of germanium. They are:

Garlic	754 ppm
Ginseng	320 ppm
Sushi	262 ppm
Sanzukon	257 ppm
Waternut	239 ppm
Comfrey	152 ppm
Boxthorn seed	124 ppm

Wisteria knob	108 ppm
Gromwell	88 ppm
Aloe	77 ppm
Chlorella	76 ppm
Bandai udo	72 ppm
Pearl barley	50 ppm

The article, "Germanium-132 (Ge-132): Homeostatic Normalizer and Immunostimulant, a Review of Its Preventive and Therapeutic Efficacy" by Parris M. Kidd, Ph.D. (*International Clinical Nutrition Review*, 7:11-20, January 1987) reports that the type of germanium in garlic has immunity-enhancing effects which correlate closely with interferon production. Interferon is a substance that is produced by cells infected with a virus and has the ability to inhibit viral growth. Germanium is one of those substances thought to stimulate the body to produce its own interferon. Germanium also "normalizes T-lymphocyte and B-lymphocyte function, natural killer cell (NK) proliferation, antibody-dependent cellular cytotoxicity, and proliferation of anti-generating cells, all of which effects could stem from its ability to stimulate interferon prodcution," writes Dr. Kidd.

Dr. Kidd says that germanium markedly stimulates gamma-interferon production, both in experimental animals and in humans over a wide age range. This interferon stimulation puts garlic's germanium in a select group of true immunostimulants (others are vitamin C, vitamin E, N, N-dimethylglycine, and Coenzyme Q_{10}). Such true immunostimulants offer advantages over the cytotoxic drugs commonly used in cancer chemotherapy. They strengthen the body's resistance to stress and disease by making tissues healthier through augmenting natural immune functions.

As with the mice I witnessed being studied at the Central Research Laboratories in Hiroshima, Japan, that were better able to cope with stress after being fed aged garlic extract, a person ingesting garlic can mount a more powerful and more balanced reaction against viral infections, tumor growth, and cancer metastasis, all without the immunosuppressive effects of cytotoxic drugs.

Selenium in Garlic Works Against Cancer

As mentioned earlier, garlic is also one of the edible plants holding the highest concentration of the trace mineral selenium. This fact becomes highly relevant when you consider the work of Gerhard Schrauzer, Ph.D. at the University of California, San Diego, which supports the concept that selenium ingestion helps to prevent cancer. Discussing his presentation on selenium's anticancer action at the 1974 Symposium on Selenium-Tellurium in the Environment, held at the University of Notre Dame, Notre Dame, Indiana, Dr. Schrauzer wrote that the incidence of spontaneous breast cancer in susceptible female mice was reduced from 82 percent to 10 percent merely by adding traces of selenium to their drinking water (*Annals of Clinical Laboratory Science,* 4:6, 441-447, May 11, 1976).

The British research physician Dr. W.C. Willett and his associates studied selenium levels in blood samples taken from 111 men and women five years or less before the development of cancer. The samples form these cancer patients were compared with blood selenium samples taken from 210 cancer-free subjects who were matched for age, weight, sex, and smoking history. In their article, "Prediagnostic Serum Selenium and Risk of Cancer" (*Lancet,* volume 130, July 16, 1983), the doctors reported that the mean blood selenium level of the cancer victims was lower (0.129 mcg/ml) than that of the individuals who did not get cancer (0.136 mcg/ml). The compared blood level numbers are small but significant when you realize that we are dealing here with a microgram (mcg) which is one ten-thousandths of a gram. Statistical projection of Dr. Willett's study indicates that those people with a 0.0007 mcg/ml elevation of their serum selenium levels have a 5.5 reduced risk of developing cancer. Supplementing with aged garlic extract, therefore, could well be a viable food source for consuming the required amount of selenium to elevate one's blood level of this anticancer mineral.

Laboratory Proof of Anticancer Factors in Aged Garlic Liquid

Using liquid aged garlic extract as the exclusive therapeutic agent, immunologist Benjamin Lau, M.D., Ph.D., Professor of Microbiology at Loma Linda University School of Medicine, has reported the cure of mouse tumors. In his published paper, "Superiority of Intralesional Immunotherapy with *Corynebacterium parvum* and *Allium sativum* in Control of Murine Transitional Cell Carcinoma" (*The Journal of Urology,* 136: 701-705, September 1986), Dr. Lau deals with a common form of cancer in mice (the murine subfamily). Transitional cell carcinoma involves the superficial layers of the bladder and has a high frequency of recurrence not only in murinae but also in homo sapiens (mankind). After surgery, recurrence rates of bladder cancer may amount to 60 or 70 percent; while chemotherapy can reduce the cancer recurrence in mice and humans to 40 or 50 percent.

In recent years, bacillus Calmette-Guerin (BCG) vaccine has been used to further cut down significantly on recurrence rates of this transitional cell carcinoma. Despite its encouraging results, BCG does have limitations. These drawbacks include irritation to the bladder, danger of systemic infection, potential generalized toxicity, and occasionally, even more serious complications. Such drawbacks have prompted Dr. Lau and his associates to evaluate other forms of immunotherapy.

In his published paper, Dr. Lau reported that his researchers tested four substances for therapeutic effects on mouse bladder cancer: (1) BCG; (2) a killed vaccine of *Corneybacterium parvum* (CP); (3) keyhole limpet hemacyanin (KLH); and (4) *Allium sativum* (AS) supplied as liquid, aged, deodorized garlic extract furnished by a Japanese pharmaceutical company. CP and AS were more effective than BCG and KLH in stopping the cancer growth. Five consecutive treatments with CP or garlic completely terminated the growth of cancer while the same number of treatments with BCG and KLH only reduced the growth about 50 percent.

Dr. Lau states that both BCG and CP have been used in cancer therapy in the prior two decades with inconsistent and often disappointing results. His work during the past ten years has identified some repeated problems with administration of BCG or CP immuotherapy. First, the therapy was prescribed when the tumor was too large. Second, the agents have been given by the wrong routes (the intravenous route rather than the intralesional route is most often used). Third, the dosages applied were often too high, leading to severe toxicity.

He and his associates have shown that in order for immunotherapy to work, the immune stimulant—known in medicine as biological response modifier (BRM)—must come in direct contact with the tumor cells. In the case of bladder cancer, this is accomplished with ease. The advantage of immunotherapy in bladder cancer lies in being able to put the BRM directly into the bladder (injecting it intralesionally). Dr. Lau believes that this approach can also be employed in other cancers such as those found in the rectum, uterine cervix, mouth, nose, and prostate, since the BRM can be either delivered or injected directly into the tumor sites.

Garlic was included as an immunotherapeutic agent in Dr. Lau's current mouse bladder tumor study because of a published 1958 paper by Drs. A.S. Weisberger and J. Pensky, "Tumor Inhibition by a Sulfhydryl-blocking Agent Related to an Active Principle of Garlic (*Allium sativum*)" (*Cancer Research,* 32:551, 1975), which reported inhibition of tumor growth when garlic was pre-incubated with tumor cells and then injected into animals. Thus garlic was combined with tumor cells. After their incubation together, the garlic-tumor culture was injected into various sites in an animal's body. Ordinarily, when cancer cells are injected into animals they grow well and produce tumors. Not so here when garlic was involved. Instead, complete inhibition of tumor growth occurred. The researchers could not explain their findings then but thought that garlic had a direct toxicity against tumor cells.

Dr. Lau believes differently. He thinks that the tumor inhibition occurred because of white blood cell stimulation and close contact between the garlic BRM and tumor cells. His current intralesional injection work confirms this hypothesis. For instance, near the conclusion of his September 1986 garlic intralesional immunotherapy paper, Dr. Lau writes:

In the present study, *Allium sativum* [AS] was shown to elicit macrophages and lymphocytes leading to cytotoxic destruction of tumor cells. It is possible that extract of AS played a dual role, inactivating sufhydryl compounds of tumor cells on the one hand and stimulating macrophages and lymphocytes on the other.

A more recent paper written by Dr. Lau, "Superiority of Intravesical Immunotherapy with Corynebacterium Parvum and Allium Sativum in Control of Murine Bladder Cancer" (*The Journal of Urology*, 137:359-362, February 1987), reports that 25 mg of aged garlic extract (AS) was advantageous in curing bladder cancer in mice when administered intravesically [the tumor grew in tiny blisters created in the bladder by electrocautery and is the manner by which the tumor was induced]. Here Dr. Lau wrote:

AS, or extract of garlic, is rich in sulfur and sulfide-containing compounds.... It is possible that AS has a dual mode of action, inactivating sulfhydryl compounds of tumor cells on the one hand and stimulating macrophages and lymphocytes on the other.... In our laboratory we have observed in vitro [in the testube] enhancement of splenic phagocytic function and natural killer cell activity associated with *Corynebacterium parvum* and AS immunotherapy.

In 1986 this immunologist also published two papers on the antimicrobial effects of garlic. His June 1986 paper in *Current Microbiology* showed that *Allium sativum* inhibits the growth of *Coccidioides immitis,* an opportunitistic fungus which inflicts itself on patients with AIDS. In another paper published in the September 1986 issue of *Antimicrobial Agents and Chemotherapy,* Dr. Lau pointed out that garlic inhibits lipid synthesis by *Candida albicans,* a common yeast organism to be discussed later in this book, in the section on chronic, generalized candidiasis (The Yeast Syndrome).

Garlic Chemical May Prevent Colon Cancer

A release from the Associated Press, dated March 25, 1986, headlined studies presented to the American Cancer Society seminar for science writers at Daytona Beach, Florida. Dr. Michael Wargovich, assistant professor of cell biology and assistant cell biologist at the University of Texas System Cancer Center and M.D. Anderson Hospital and Tumor Institute in Houston, said that a garlic sulfur compound may prevent colon cancer. Dially sulfide, the odorous allicin breakdown product that occurs when raw clove garlic is crushed and exposed to the air, was found in animal research to inhibit the early cell changes associated with colon cancer. The substance is now being tested for a direct link to preventing colon cancer in mice.

During his interview, Dr. Wargovich explained that the garlic breakdown substance was given to animals before they were exposed to a potent cancer-causing agent, and they failed to get cancer. It is now being tested further for a direct link to preventing colon cancer in mice and eventually humans.

Dr. Wargovich said he can't yet recommend whether people should take aged garlic extract to prevent colon cancer. In its purified form, diallyl sulfide hasn't been tested for side effects. However, he added, garlic itself reduces blood fats and cholesterol, both factors in heart disease, and "I don't think eating garlic is going to cause any sort of harm."

Successful Garlic Treatment of Cancer in China

Another more recent Associated Press release headlined its story: "Garlic Keeps Cancer Away, Chinese Say." In Peking, researchers have found the everyday staple of the Chinese diet, whole clove garlic, is an effective anticancer agent because it blocks the formation of nitrosamine, a strong carcinogen.

Since 1983, investigators at Shangdon Province Medical College, Jinan Chemical Research Institute, and Peking Medical College, all located in Peking, China, have been studying the use of raw garlic to prevent nitrosamine carcinogenesis. In 1987, they proved that garlic's nutritional components control nitrosamine by preventing the growth of the molds and germs which synthesize it as well as blocking their destructive chemical activities. Another authoritative source says the same thing. Actively engaged in research with a special interest in the relationship of nutrition and cancer, John Wu, M.D., retired faculty member of the Department of Pathology at the College of Physicians and Surgeons of Columbia University, New York City, also reports on garlic as a cancer preventive. In a letter to the author, Dr. Wu advises, "Residents of Gangsan County in China who regularly consume 20 grams of garlic a day have a gastric cancer mortality of only 3.45 per 100,000 [population] whereas residents of the neighboring Quixia county who rarely eat any garlic have a gastric cancer mortality rate of 40 per 100,000.

"Gangshan county residents who eat large amounts of garlic have lower concentrations of nitrite in their gastric juice [nitrite is a carcinogen] than those in Quixia county," continued Dr. Wu. "Garlic reduces the nitrite concentration by inhibiting the growth of bacteria which are capable of converting nitrate into nitrite. However, since it is known that nitrites are present in vegetables, meat, and even tap water, simple inhibition of nitrate conversion is inadequate. My experiments have shown that the crucial step is further blocking of the reaction of nitrite with amines that otherwise leads to the formation of nitrosamine, a potent carcinogen."

Dr. Wu suggests that garlic as a nontoxic edible product can effectively block this nitrosamine reaction, producing a significant reduction in cancer mortality. The odorless garlic extract, taken as a food supplement, thus finds use as preventive, anticarcinogenic dietary product. He adds, "Liver sections of rats treated with sodium nitrite, aminopyrine, and garlic extract confirm that addition of garlic prevents the necrotic lesions indicative of nitrosamine formation and carcinogenesis."

Also, pathologist Dr. John Wu continues, "Even more exciting results have been obtained in another series of experiments in which sarcoma 180 ascites cells transplanted into susceptible mice either failed to produce tumors when garlic extract was mixed with the cells or, if greater numbers of ascites cells were injected, produced tumors which regressed within one month when drinking water was also supplemented with garlic extract. I believe that the observed effects of garlic extract [to prevent cancer] are extremely promising and worthy of further exploration," his letter concludes.

The Yeast Syndrome (Candidiasis)

Candida albicans is a yeast organism growing in and on our bodies. It is normally controlled by our immune defenses and by the usual bacterial flora present in everyone's intestinal tract. But when ecological change takes place in one's internal environment, helpful bacteria decrease and immune response becomes depressed. Then the condition known as chronic, generalized candidiasis (The Yeast Syndrome) arises. Nothing remains to stop *C. albicans* from producing a number of devastating toxins which destroy the host person's health.

From the mouth to the anus and down to the toes, this fungus gives rise to a syndrome—the signs and symptoms of candidiasis disease. The Yeast Syndrome may involve abdominal pain, menstrual pain, weakness, depression, mental disorientation, earache, fatigue, infertility, lost sex drive, persistent cough, recurrent vaginitis, skin irritation, constipation, diarrhea, bloating, heartburn, migraine headache, allergic reaction, anxiety, asthma, athlete's foot, and a lot more trouble. Physician members of the American Academy of Environmental Medicine who specialize in treatment of The Yeast Syndrome estimate that it strikes every third person around the world. As many as 15 percent of all adult men, 20 percent of all children, and 70 percent of all adult women have it as an underlying (subclinical) illness or as an active and spreading disease.

An Amazing Case History of Conquering Candidiasis

Living in a trailer park around Mt. Pinos, California, Lola thatcher, now 37 years old, has been a victim of candidiasis for the past eight years. She has experienced nearly all of the symptoms mentioned above as a result of this condition. The Yeast Syndrome caused her to be allergic to such a variety of common household items that her allergist classified the woman as a "universal reactor." Indeed, Mrs. Thatcher's allergy response was ready to react like a bomb to any substance to which her immune system took exception.

So extreme was Mrs. Thatcher's hypersensitivity, she had to wear only clothing made of cotton or other natural fabrics; her drinking water was distilled; aluminum foil covered the walls in her home rather than paint or wallpaper paste; her television, set at a permanently high volume to be heard through the window, was positioned outside the house; since the unfortunate woman was forced to stay away from people except for her husband and children, the nearest neighbor lived two miles away. She rode in an automobile less than a dozen times during this eight-year period of universal allergy reaction. And when she did ride, her breathing needed to be supported with an oxygen tank and special filter.

She suffered from insomnia; exhaustion let her perform very few homemaker chores. She had intestinal parasites occasionally showing in her stool. Because of her violent allergic response to printer's ink, she could not be near printed reading materials. This prompted a group of concerned friends to join together and rewrite *The Bible* for her in pencil so that she could read something spiritual and historical.

All of this trouble came from the overgrowth of *C. albicans* in her body, which has been exceedingly difficult to dislodge.

Mrs. Thatcher has not been idle in attempting to rid herself of The Yeast Syndrome. She spent nearly $150 a month on the antiyeast drug, nystatin, which is commonly prescribed for treatment of candidiasis. She followed an organic rotation diet that allowed for megadose nutrition and the avoidance of certain foods to which her body is intolerant. She took high doses of assorted nutrients, too, but nothing seemed to do much good. Today, most of the description I have just given for Lola Thatcher has changed. Her circumstances are much improved because of a knowledgeable and empathetic woman named Nancy Burnett, a Yeast Syndrome researcher residing in Cottonwood, Arizona. Mrs. Burnett has put the candidiasis victim on a strict, mostly complex carbohdrate regimen. Mrs. Thatcher eats no meat, oils, sugar, dairy products or yeast products. Moreover, she takes a tablespoon and a half of Pines Wheat Grass Powder with each meal. Wheat grass is rich in beta carotene, which is 25 percent natural protein and high in vitamins (notably vitamin B-12), minerals, chlorophyll, and a fiber that offers therapeutic roughage without harshness. The wheat grass and aged garlic has helped to bring Mrs. Thatcher back from her unusual hypersensitivity and its associated exaggerated allergic reactions.

Even more helpful, the primary treatment against her chronic, generalized candidiasis is the eight teaspoonsful of liquid, aged, deodorized garlic extract that Nancy Burnett has made part of Lola Thatcher's daily nutrition program. Like the wheat grass, this garlic is processed from plants grown in organically pure soil, free of all pesticides, fungicides, fumigants, and other chemical agents. It is also significant to note that Lola had been allergic to cooked garlic, whereas her immune system readily accepts the aged, cold-processed liquid garlic that she swallows several times daily as a food supplement. Taking this herb in extract form each day has driven much of the pathological yeast from her body. The aged garlic extract has taken the place of the prescription drug, nystatin.

The patient's improved physical, emotional, and mental condition is amazing to witness. Nancy's combination garlic/wheat grass/dietary regimen is the definitive countervailing solution to Lola's formerly debilitating candidiasis condition.

In an interview, Lola Thatcher said, "I go to bed at 8:00 p.m. and wake up about 4:30 a.m. feeling totally refreshed rather than sick, weak, and drugged [as she once was]. My depression is gone, my eyes are clear, and each day I feel better and stronger. It used to be a real struggle to walk a quarter of a mile for my mail, now I jog thirty miles every week. For a limited time each day, I can now read printed pages—books and a newspaper—without any allergic response."

No longer does she need that antiyeast drug which had been the single, prescribed pharmaceutical antidote for her chronic, generalized candidiasis. Lola's antidote now is all natural: an enhanced raw foods diet that is supplemented with garlic extract, wheat grass, and other items acquired from the health food store rather than from the drug store.

In a letter from Lola Thatcher, dated December 7, 1987, she says.

I was so delighted with my results from the liquid aged garlic extract, I must admit I was prejudiced and much in favor of this liquid. And now capsules filled with garlic powder are working even better. Probably the liquid served a very important part of my healing in the beginning and this is a transitional period, so the powder filled capsules are doing wonderfully well for me during this new period.

My bowel movements are improved overall. I've been passing more worms again, too, for which I am very glad. I feel a little better each time they show themselves, and I get rid of them.

It has been two years since I was in an automobile. Recently I took a ride and used my oxygen for only half the time I was in the car (the first time I could breathe automobile fumes and regular air without inhaling from my oxygen tank in five-and-a-half years). I was driven to my parents house regarding some matters about my grandmother's death. Part of my grandmother's furniture became mine and was brought up to my home. In the wood was impregnated over sixty years of cigarette smoke and heavy oil-based perfume smells. Before taking my aged garlic extract, I easily would have become semiconscious from just a couple sniffs of that wood. Now it decorates my home with no health problem for me.

I used to have to hang all our mail on the clothes line to air out the smells for several days to several weeks, depending on how strong the mail's odor. But now the mail comes in the house (except that catalogues are stored outside). Even with perfume samples in them, I can read the correspondence right away. (I would have passed out before). Also, I once could not write a letter with ink because I became too spacey and tired from the fumes. Now I write all of my correspondence in ink.

I was taking ten powdered aged garlic capsules a day at first. When stress was real bad I went to as many as twenty capsules a day as well as increasing my intake of wheat grass and charcoal. Now I basically stay at twelve to sixteen garlic capsules daily and am working down to ten, except on high stress days such as Thanksgiving day holiday weekend.

However, coping with Thanksgiving wasn't any problem this past year. I remained in my parent's home celebrating the holiday with eleven family members present for over seven-and-a-half hours and did really well. I looked at all the rich, gourmet foods and desserts and didn't crave them. I brought my our own food for my immediate family and me.

I started off with the garlic capsules in mid-March 1987. It was extremely stressful for me during that time as a series of minor crises happened.

Nancy Burnett's dietary program and the deodorized garlic capsules saw me through this stress and my suffering with the Yeast Syndrome. I thank God that the aged garlic extract has been developed by the Japanese company and that it's imported into the United States.

Lola Thatcher's son, born in 1981, who has been a victim of The Yeast Syndrome since birth, is maintained by his mother on the same regimen as hers, except that he is given lesser amounts of food, garlic, wheat grass, and other nutrients. According to Mrs. Thatcher, the child is less emotionally disturbed than he was previously and has far more energy. Of course, he does complain, as most children will, about the need to eat all those vegetables which comprise the major food components of Nancy Burnett's antiyeast eating program.

"I pieced together an educational program on this yeast condition," explained Nancy Burnett during our discussions. "I learned from physicians who were treating it successfully. My program just flatout works. I teach a diet that's somewhat at odds with the present Candida Control Diet developed by Dr. John Parks Trowbridge and described in the book that he wrote with you [*The Yeast Syndrome*, Bantam Books, November 1986, available at most book stores and health food stores, or you may purchase it through the mail by sending $6.00 to New Way of Life, Inc., the publisher of this book]. I believe that the Candida Control Diet's requirement of eating all that animal protein tends to promote chemical sensitivities, so here in my Better Living Center I recommend the consumption of some grains and lots of vegetables.

"I run a series of nine, two-hour classes to provide an 18-hour course on candidiasis. Audiotapes are sold, too. All I do is teach how to eat what comes from the hand of the Creator without the adding of coloring agents, preservatives, and other manmade items. I also teach the values of exercise, good drinking water, sunlight, fresh air breathing, balance, rest, the spirit, and other wholistic things. I don't prescribe anything but just give health education," said Mrs. Burnett.

For more information about Lola Thantcher's successful regimen against The Yeast Syndrome, contact Nancy Burnett at the Better Living Center, 114 West Main, Cottonwood, Arizona 86326; telephone (602) 634-2017.

Blood Fats Reduction and Atherosclerosis Reversal

Interest in garlic for immunologist Dr. Benjamin Lau of Loma Linda University goes back six years when colleagues in research and medicine approached him to look into the validity of the herb as a medical therapeutic agent. After reviewing the literature on the subject, he and two colleagues, Moses A. Adetumbi, M.A. of the Department of Microbiology, School of Medicine, and Albert Sanchez, D.P.H., of the Department of Nutrition, School of Health, both of Loma Linda University, researched and published "Garlic and Atherosclerosis: a Review" (*Nutrition Research*, January/February 1983). They cited 49 medical journal articles on laboratory and/or clinical investigations of garlic that relate to fat metabolism and hardening of the arteries. The data suggest that garlic is of value in both prevention and treatment of cardiovascular diseases. From every corner of the world, Dr. Lau has received over 2,000 requests for reprints of this, his first paper on the therapeutic uses of garlic.

Clinical studies uncovered by the literature search by Lau, Adetumbi, and Sanchez show that garlic's components lower elevated serum cholesterol and triglyceride levels, improve the very low density lipoproteins (VLDL) to high density lipoproteins (HDL) blood lipoprotein ratio, affect blood coagulation parameters, and are of value in the prevention or treatment of diseases arising from hardening of the arteries. Their literature search was divided into two sections, one devoted to animal experiments and the other to studies on people. I shall report on the animal investigations first.

Garlic's Vascular Benefits Shown by Laboratory Animals

K.T. Augusti and P.T. Mathew, reporting in "Lipid Lowering Effect of Allicin (Diallyl Disulphide-oxide) on Long Term Feeding to Normal Rats" (Experientia, 30:468-470, 1974), fed animals a regular laboratory diet for two months and compared them to those supplemented daily with 100 mg/kg of allicin extracted from garlic. The allicin-fed group showed statistically significant reductions in total serum lipids, phospholipids, and cholesterol as compared to the control group.

Arun Bordia and his coworkers, reporting in "The Protective Action of Essential Oils of Onion and Garlic in Cholesterol-Fed Rabbits" (Atherosclerosis, 22:103-109, 1975), made observations similar to Augusti and Mathew. Bordia's group compared the effect of garlic oil with a commercially available generic antilipidemic (blood-fat lowering) agent called clofibrate. The outcome of this study indicated that in those laboratory animals fed a cholesterol-supplemented diet, the decreases in blood cholesterol associated with ingestion of garlic were much better statistically than with clofibrate.

Again, Arun Bordia and S.K. Verma, in an article, "Effect of Garlic on the Reversibility of Experimental Atherosclerosis" (Indian Heart Journal, 30:47-50, 1978), and in their second article on this subject, "Effect of Garlic Feeding on Regression of Experimental

Atherosclerosis in Rabbits" (*Artery*, 7:428-437, 1980), reported two more studies in which animals were supplemented with a diet consisting of .5g/kg cholesterol for three months. The test animals were then divided into two groups. One half of the animals were supplemented by the investigators with freeze-dried garlic. Blood analysis revealed this supplemented group had increased levels of "good" HDL with concurrent decreases in low density lipoproteins (LDL) and VLDL levels. (This "good" HDL fraction of blood lipids has been associated with lowered incidence of heart disease, primarily due to its inhibitory effect on LDL uptake by the arterial walls and its assistance in transporting cholesterol to the liver where it is catabolized or discarded from the body.)

R.C. Jain, reporting in "Onion and Garlic in Experimental Cholesterol-Induced Atherosclerosis" (*Indian Journal of Medicine and Research*, 64:1509-1515, 1976), compared the effect of garlic and onion on rabbits fed a diet high in cholesterol. The group of animals supplemented with garlic showed insignificant rises in blood cholesterol as compared to elevated blood cholesterol in the onion-supplemented animals and a very high blood cholesterol in the non-supplemented animals. Jain concluded that garlic lowers serum cholesterol.

A second study carried out by R.C. Jain and D.B. Konar, "Effect of Garlic Oil in Experimental Cholesterol Atherosclerosis" (*Atherosclerosis*, 29:125-129, 1978), showed that the cholesterol-lowering effect of garlic is dose-related. The more garlic powder extract fed the rabbits daily, the greater the effect. These rabbits had a 30 percent reduction in serum cholesterol when aged garlic extract comprised about 2 percent of the animals' high-cholesterol, atherosclerosis-promoting diet.

M.L.W. Chang and M.A. Johnson, reporting in "Effect of Garlic on Carbohydrate Metabolism and Lipid Synthesis in Rats" (*Journal of Nutrition*, 110:931-936, 1980), gave rats a diet containing one percent cholesterol and sucrose. Then the researchers decreased serum total fat in the animals by feeding them the equivelant of five grams of fresh garlic bulbs per day for seven days.

Forty more animal studies could be reported here, all with

results similar to those described above. In summary, other investigators support the cited findings in studies of experimental hardening of the arteries that supplementation of laboratory animals' diets with aged garlic extract decreases cholesterol and phospholipids. Such decrease results in a lower degree of atherosclerosis for the animals, as confirmed by fewer atheromatous lesions being found on autopsy.

Beneficial Effects of Garlic on Atherosclerosis in People

Most of the clinical studies evaluating the effects of garlic on blood fats, cholesterol, atheromatous lesions, and generalized atherosclerosis in human subjects have been carried out in India. For example, an epidemiological study comparing three populations with different dietary habits was reported by G.S. Sainani and his associates in their paper, "Effect of Dietary Garlic and Onion on Serum Lipid Profile in Jain Community" (*Indian Journal of Medical Research*, 69:776-780, 1979). Vegeterians in the Jain community of India were matched for age, sex, weight, and social status. They consisted of those who consumed onion and garlic: (a) in liberal amounts, (b) in small amounts, or (c) not at all. The liberal garlic consumers had the lowest level of serum cholesterol and serum triglycerides. Total abstainers showed the highest level. Sainani's study is significant because the subjects chosen had similar daily diets in regards to calories, fat, and carbohydrate intake. Their only dietary difference was in the eating of onion and garlic.

Also the Jain community population differed in their blood coagulation parameters. The group with total abstinence from the allium family of herbs had significantly higher plasma fibrinogen, shorter clotting time, poorer fibrinolytic activity, and were more inclined to form blood vessel blockage than the other two groups.

Writing in "Hypocholesterolaemic Effect of Garlic *Allium sativum*" (*Indian Journal of Experimental Biology*, 15:489-490, 1977), K.T. Augusti reported that he lowered the serum cholesterol in five patients by giving them garlic juice to drink once a day for two months. When the garlic drinking stopped, in two months their blood cholesterol increased again to pretreatment levels. In their 1987 paper published in *Nutrition Research* (volume 7, pages 139-149), Benjamin H.S. Lau, M.D., Ph.D., Fred Lam, M.D., and Rebekah Wang-Cheng, M.D. of the Department of Microbiology and Medicine, School of Medicine, Loma Linda University described the "Effect of an Odor-Modified Garlic Preparation on Blood Lipids." The three physicians wrote:

The effect of an odor-modified liquid garlic extract on blood lipids was evaluated in human subjects over a six month period. Lowering of cholesterol, triglycerides, low density and very low density lipoproteins (LDL/VLDL) with rise of high density lipoprotein (HDL) was observed in the majority of subjects who took garlic extract; the effect was clearly more significant than with subjects taking placebo. Garlic extract did not significantly influence the levels of cholesterol and triglycerides in subjects whose initial cholesterol levels were relatively low. Of special interest was the initial rise of cholesterol, triglycerides, and LDL/VLDL with garlic supplementation, suggesting possible mobilization of tissue lipids into the circulation during this phase of garlic ingestion. This study confirms previous reports of lowering cholesterol and triglycerides using various garlic preparations. Furthermore, it suggests that odor-modified garlic extract may be used in conjunction with dietary modification for control of hyperlipidemia [elevated blood fats].

Our study with this commercial product from Japan [aged, deodorized garlic, referred to as 'odor-modified garlic,' prepared from pure garlic bulbs by a cold-aging process which removes the pungent odor but still retains its active components] confirms that odorless garlic extract is indeed effective in lowering cholesterol and triglycerides in the majority of human subjects.

(Note: For a reprint of this paper or any other scientific investigation published by Dr. Lau and his associates, send a large-size, self-addressed envelope with postage for three ounces of mail to Benjamin H.S. Lau, M.D., Ph.D., P.O. Box 1821, Loma Linda,

California 92354 U.S.A.)

Arun Bordia, reporting in "Effect of Garlic on Blood Lipids in Patients with Coronary Heart Disease" (American Journal of Clinical Nutrition, 30:1380-1381, 1977), studied the effect of garlic on lipoproteins in 62 heart attack patients. These patients were divided into two groups. The first group was placed on garlic and the second group was not, merely serving as a control. Lipoproteins remained at constant levels in the control group but showed a steady decrease of LDL and VLDL accompanied by a progressive rise of HDL in the garlic group.

More Generalized Studies of Effects on Human Health

Arun Bordia, also reporting in "Effect of Garlic on Human Platelet Aggregation in Vitro" (Atherosclerosis, 30:355-360, 1978), said that the oral administration of aged garlic extract inhibited thrombus formation associated with platelet aggregation.

This same effect of refined and deodorized extract of garlic was studied by three independent groups of scientists in England, Japan, and India. These investigators demonstrated that aged garlic extract inhibited in vitro platelet aggregation induced by epinephrine or collagen, and that the extent of the beneficial effect was determined by how much garlic was taken.

The largest combined group of studies ever conducted on the healing powers of garlic are ongoing right now, in Japan. In one investigation, medical researchers are examining the herb's effects as a refined, aged, deodorized extract on nearly 150 patients at 25 hospitals nationwide. Dr. Tohru Fuwa, of Hiroshima University, director of this study, has already shown that the aged garlic extract offers significant improvements in treating heart, liver, digestive, and neurologic diseases, as well as other ailments.

According to Dr. Fuwa, another study already completed on 131 patients at the Hiroshima University Hospital and eight other hospitals pointed up that garlic extract reduced symptoms and restored health in 110 cases of subclinical illness and outright disease. More than 50 percent of all the patients reported marked improvement in neurologic, digestive, heart, and liver ailments. In addition, Dr. Fuwa says that the garlic extract is effective in treating subjective disorders such as fatigue, stiffness, chills, and anorexia. It is a primary remedy for chronic fatigue syndrome from Epstein-Barr virus and cytomegalovirus, which are sweeping industrialized countries.

Garlic Reversal of Hypertension

Attributing his current teenage-level blood pressure to deodorized, aged garlic extract, Carleton Ronkowsky of Torrance, California acknowledges that normal health wasn't always his good fortune. Three years ago, this chief accountant at a major aerospace corporation underwent a routine company physical. He was much overweight then, and the physician found Ronkowsky's blood pressure was elevated to the dangerous level of 190/100—potentially a candidate for heart attack.

The industrial physician prescribed the beta blocking drug, Inderol™, to bring down Ronkowsky's blood pressure, and Zaroxolyn™ as a diuretic. It appeared that the patient would have to be on these drugs the rest of his life. He also followed doctor's orders by modifying his diet with more fruit and raw vegetables, and agreed to do some exercise (by mowing his lawn on Saturday mornings).

Reading about the value of raw garlic as a natural treatment for hypertension, Ronkowsky opted to take garlic oil perles so that he wouldn't have odoriferous breath. He swallowed the perles along with his medication. On the label it said that garlic oil was odorless, but his wife and friends told him differently. He learned that he carried the smell of garlic with him all the time. His conclusion was that this nutritional supplement wasn't for him. It caused him to stink!

In a health food store at Mammoth Lake, California one day, the accountant saw an attractive garlic food supplement display and commented on it to the store's proprietor. But he refused the proprietor's proffered trial samples of aged garlic extract in encapsulated powder form. Still, the store owner was insistent, and finally Ronkowsky accepted the free samples.

A few days later during a lunch break, he took four capsules with water and, much to his surprise none of his fellow workers made the usual garlic odor jokes that afternoon. He did not seem to smell. The real test came that evening when he arrived home and kissed his wife and she failed to turn up her nose. The next day was a repeat performance with the same result. "Eureka!" declared Carleton Ronkowsky. "I've found garlic that's really deodorized."

He began religiously to take the aged garlic extract—nine capsules a day in a divided dose of three at each meal. A month later he checked his own blood pressure with a home blood pressure testing device. Ronkowsky found his hypertension much reduced, so he cut the daily dosage of his two medications to just half and kept up his garlic intake. In another month his blood pressure was down to 140/90, and the patient cut back his medicines again to just one-quarter dose. At the end of a third month on deodorized garlic, he recorded his blood pressure at 127/80. Ronkowsky stopped taking the prescribed medication altogether and just relied on aged garlic extract to keep his blood pressure normal. It stayed that way.

At his semi-annual checkup with the industrial physician, Ronkowsky was found to have blood pressure better than "normal" for his age group. The doctor immediately credited the patient's success to the prescription medicines. The doctor said, "Carleton, you have the blood pressure of a teeanger!" At this point Ronkowsky confessed that he had been taking capsules of aged garlic extract. With a broad grin, the company physician said, "Whatever you're doing, keep doing it."

Today, Ronkowsky has permanently left the ranks of 50 million Americans suffering from hypertension. He remains in this enviable position because his garlic food supplement has become a regular part of his dietary intake.

Garlic Cures Acute and Chronic Ear Infections

Melissa Staie, the baby daughter of Cynthia Staie who lives in White Fish, Montana, was ill with a chronic ear infection. Mrs. Staie first took the child to her family physician, and then she consulted an otolaryngtolgist (ear specialist) whom he recommended. The two doctors finally decided that the little girl needed an ear operation. While the baby was on the hospital operating table in preparation for surgery, her anesthesiologist discovered that he could not put his tiny patient under anesthesia. It would endanger her life. Consequently, the ear surgeon declared that there was nothing more he and the hospital's staff could do for Melissa.

In desperation, Mrs. Staie took the baby to a homeopathic physician who prescribed deodorized, aged, liquid garlic extract as an ear drop and for oral administration. Within two days Melissa's ear infection disappeared. The baby girl has not required medical attention to her ear since.

Joshua, the baby son of Salt Lake City resident Mary Ledbetter, periodically developed a painful right ear problem. It was an acute infection which temporarily cleared with the use of antibiotics but chronically returned. One such infection persisted for seven months. Antibiotics prescribed by the child's pediatrician proved ineffective against it, and many nights Joshua would awaken and cry nonstop. No other solution for the acute ear infection seemed available except for the doctor to insert a tube in the ear to drain away the infection. Mrs. Ledbetter didn't want such surgical-type treatment for her little boy.

Discussing the child's ear problem with a neighbor, Mary learned that processed, liquid, aged garlic was a viable remedy for acute and chronic ear infections. She gave little Joshua a teaspoonful a day of aged garlic extract by mouth. She also bathed the interior of his ear with three or four drops of the extract. Every few days she washed his ear with a solution of one-half distilled water and one-half apple cider vinegar.

The result? The acute infection disappeared and its residual chronicity became less and less frequent. Within four months the infection disappeared completely and has not returned in four years. Today, Joshua, now age six, is in excellent health and continues to stay with the remedy that saved him from an ear operation—aged garlic extract in liquid form.

Garlic Tablets Balance a Diabetic's Insulin Needs

Bernadette Wisner of South Belgrave, Australia is the mother of an 18-year-old daughter who is an insulin-dependent diabetic. "Due to her age and lifestyle," writes Mrs. Wisner, "she found it difficult to sometimes control her condition with just one insulin injection a day. The endocrinologist warned her that if her high blood glucose readings did not come down, the only solution was to take injections twice a day, morning and night.

"My daughter did not want this double stick and became quite upset. She pointed out that she already was as close to a human pincushion as one can get. She has been a diabetic for four years and tried but didn't always succeed with her diabetic diet," said the sympathetic mother. "I mentioned this to our chemist [pharmacist], who then suggested that she try using garlic tablets which had been deodorized. After one week on this aged garlic extract (just one in the morning and one in the evening), my daughter's blood glucose readings came down and have stayed down for the past eight months. She remains on the garlic tablets to make sure that her insulin needs remain in balance."

The Healing Powers of Garlic in Ileitis

Journalist Steven Parker of Santa Monica, California, now nearly 40 years old, suffered for 15 years with ileitis, an inflammation of the lower portion of the small bowel. Ileitis is often chronic and can require surgery to produce a cure.

"At the ages of both 12 and 17 I underwent major abdominal surgical resections, and was resigned to a life of almost constant intestinal pain, severely decreased energy, very drastic mood changes, and a recurring rash on my face," wrote Parker in a letter for publication.

Every day for 15 years the young man took, in varying doses, aspirin, azulfidine, and cortisone (prednisone). The combination of all these drugs produced an anti-inflammatory and antibiotic action to combat his ileitis, but they were accompanied by awful side effects. Then an informed friend told Parker that purified liquid, aged garlic extract might be used as an effective substitute for the different medications. He tried it.

"I am happy to report that since I started taking the garlic I have not been sidelined for even one day with an ileitis attack [that's eight years ago]! I normally take two of the liquid capsules every morning," wrote Parker. "I eat and drink what I please, when I please, with no restrictions. On days when I do feel a bit weak or ill-tempered (these are my characteristic signs of an impending ileitis attack), I increase my aged garlic extract dosage to six or ten capsules for a day or so, and then go back to my two-a-day without having to experience a day of illness.

"I was hopeful and confident that one day I would find the 'perfect' medicine for this disease, considered life-long and incurable by all of the top medical experts. It seems I have found my cure in as simple and inexpensive a health food store product as aged garlic extract. This is the longest period I have gone in 15 years without an ileitis attack. I am ever grateful and make the product an integral part of my dietary intake."

Garlic as a Detoxifier in Systemic Lupus Erythematosus

Forty-two -year-old Albert Lowenstein of Los Angeles had just completed a 19-month, three-drug therapy program for tuberculosis. During this time his chief complaints were a skin rash on the face, extreme fatigue, and generalized joint pains, all of which continued after the program's completion. He also ran a low-grade, intermittent fever of 99.8 degrees F. The symptoms seemed unrelated to tuberculosis, which the doctors said was under good control.

"I then began experiencing more severe joint pain on my left side as well as up and down my spine. Headaches set in along with severe depression, and I had definite sensitivity to the sun," Lowenstein explained. "Within six months I was diagnosed by one of the many medical specialists I finally consulted for these assorted discomforts as having systemic lupus erythematosus. Another specialist warned that I was in for severe disability, so much so that I wouldn't be able to work anymore."

Systemic lupus erythematosus is a bizarre disease, related to rheumatoid arthritis, which attacks various parts of the body. The cause is unknown but is thought to come from a latent virus that lies dormant until its destructive effects are triggered by sunlight, another infection, some chemical, or by other unidentifiable agents. This is an autoimmune disease in which the body's tissues are attacked by its own immune system cells, whose normal function is to fight off foreign invaders.

"Rather than start another toxic drug therapy program for treating my lupus," continued Al Lowenstein, "I began treatment with a homeopathic physician. This M.D. put me on a healthy diet, various vitamins and herbs, and a detoxifiying program. The main detoxifying herbal remedy he prescribed was aged garlic extract in liquid form. I also went on periodic juice fasts with liquid deodorized garlic added to the juice to speed up the process of detoxfication.

"Let me assure you that this remedy works. Aged, deodorized garlic is truly nature's healer. Slowly my symptoms began to disappear," said Lowenstein. "The rash on my face went first, losing its butterfly-shaped appearance that had spread across my nose and cheeks. Inside of a year of the treatment, my fever had disappeared and body temperature remained a normal 98.6 degrees F. Ninety percent of my chronic joint pain was gone, and no problem with the sun remained. It's three years now since I first was diagnosed as having lupus. Even though to this day my blood tests still show slightly positive for the disease, I am feeling just fine. Aged garlic extract in the liquid form remains very much a part of my daily life. It's the one remedy that solved my life-threatening disease of systemic lupus erythematosus. I am grateful that this medicinal food supplement remains available to me. I wouldn't want to be without it."

For Depression, Sports Injuries, and Other Uses

Naturopath and sports psychologist Dr. Ritchi Morris is an ardent prescriber of aged garlic extract in all its forms. Dr. Morris, who is Director of Employee Assistance Resource Services of Ardsley, New York, combines the odor-modified garlic with other nutritional remedies such as vitamin C, ginseng, germanium, and N,N-Dimethyglycine (DMG). He uses these nutrient combinations in the treatment of patients clinically exhibiting depressive personalities. He says that the nutrients reduce the frequency and intensity of his patients' depressions.

"When I eliminated the aged garlic extract unbeknownst to the patients," added Dr. Morris, "the frequency and intensity of depression increased slightly. And when I placed the garlic back into their regimen, the depression's frequency and intensity reduced again.

"As a pain reliever in sports injuries, aged garlic extract works well. I've had much success with professional athletes on teams such as the New York Giants, Rangers, Arrows, Nets, Knicks, Yankees, and Olympians, as well as for myself as a competing powerlifter," says Morris. "I've found that when the garlic food supplement is taken after the workouts/contests/games it seems to prevent edema and the buildup of lactic acids in the athletes' cooling-down muscles. In the weightlifting arena, it has been particularly effective in helping us weightlifters to 'make weight' for our respective weight class. Garlic food supplement appears to act in two capacities: (a) as a mild diuretic; (b) as an aid in breaking down the fats and flushing them out of the body. •

"Lastly, and perhaps most importantly, it bolsters the immune system to foritfy it against all of the stress of competition and life. As the wellness of the athlete and worker is paramount, you can see the essential role for aged garlic extract," states the naturopath/psychologist.

Effectiveness of Externally Applied Liquid Deodorized Garlic

External applications of aged garlic extract in liquid form are reported by some practitioners and medical consumers alike to have been exceedingly effective in certain health problems. These externally applied remedies are used in conjunction with the oral intake of aged garlic extract in any of its forms: tablets, capsules, or liquid. Many of the following tips for the external application of garlic come from *The Khoe Newsletter,* written by Willem H. Khoe, M.D., Ph.D., D.Sc., D.Ac. of Las Vegas, Nevada, but most of the accounts are strictly anecdotal and have not been published in any clinical journal articles. It is solely the reader's responsibility to determine if treatment procedures described here are appropriate. The publisher and author, as discussed in the disclaimer at the beginning of this book, in no way assume responsibility for what already has been described or for what is to be presented now.

FOR THE RELIEF OF ACUTE CONJUNCTIVITIS: Fill an eye cup nearly to the top with distilled water. Add two drops of liquid aged garlic extract. Bathe the eye having acute conjuctivitis with the solution. You should feel immediate relief.

FOR THE TREATMENT OF AN EYE INFECTION: Mix one drop of liquid aged garlic extract with four drops of distilled water and apply as eye drops.

FOR THE TREATMENT OF AN EAR BACTERIAL OR FUNGUS INFECTION: Into the infected ear: For children, insert two or three drops of liquid aged garlic extract; for adults, insert five or six drops. Insertion may be assured by holding the liquid in place with a wisp of cotton. Do this twice a day. Wash out the ear each time before inserting a fresh application of garlic, using a mixture of apple cider vinegar and water.

FOR SINUSITIS: Dilute liquid garlic with distilled water in a one to one ratio. Have the individual recline and atomize the resultant solution into each of his nostrils. Then he should bend over with the head between his knees for 45 seconds, return to a standing position, hold the nostrils closed for 30 seconds, and then gently blow the nose. The sinus passages should clear and breathing become easy.

FOR NOSE INFECTION: Apply liquid garlic extract directly to the nasal passages with cotton swabs or atomize.

FOR MOUTH INFECTION: Apply aged garlic liquid extract directly into the mouth and swirl it around for a lengthy period, as if it is a mouth wash. Don't waste the costly solution, but swallow it for generalized internal benefits.

FOR SORE THROAT: Using the garlic extract in liquid form, gargle for 30 to 45 seconds. Swallow the liquid. Repeat the gargling every 45 minutes as necessary.

FOR TREATMENT OF LARYNGITIS: Do the same as for sore throat.

FOR BRONCHITIS OR ASTHMA: Dilute one tablespoonful of aged garlic liquid extract with three tablespoonsful of distilled water and atomize the solution into the lungs.

FOR A BAD COUGH: Well down into the throat, squirt liquid aged garlic extract each time that you must cough. Repeat the process until you have used up a day's full dispenser bottle.

FOR THE TREATMENT OF INFLUENZA VIRUS: Cut up two whole grapefruits with the skin and all; put the pieces in water and boil for twenty minutes. Let the mixutre stand and when cooled to lukewarm, add four tablespoonsful of liquid aged garlic extract. Drink the solution all at once or within 40 minutes. Continue using this drink for two days. Also take 10 to 15 capsules of the liquid garlic with 6000 mg of vitamin C in four divided doses.

FOR DETOXIFICATION OF THE COLON: Dilute one tablespoonful of liquid aged garlic extract with three tablespoonsful of warm water (at body temperature of about 42 degrees C) and apply as an enema.

FOR VAGINAL YEAST INFECTION: Make a solution as for detoxification (above) and use it for douching twice a day for at least three days. Also swallow nine capusles of the liquid aged garlic extract daily for a minimum of three days. Start the oral administation at the same time that you begin the douching.

FOR TREATMENT OF HEMORRHOIDS OR RECTAL ITCH: Directly and gently apply aged garlic liquid extract to the hemorrhoidal area, using cotton-tipped swabs. For more severe hemorrhoids apply as much as a bottle of the liquid garlic a day. Also fill one gelatin capsule with the liquid garlic and insert into the anus.

FOR PIN WORMS IN A CHILD: Fill one gelatin capsule half with water and half with liquid aged garlic extract. Insert the filled capsule into the child's rectum while he or she is asleep.

FOR TREATMENT OF ACNE OR PIMPLES: Before retiring for the night, apply liquid aged garlic extract directly to the skin lesions, accompanied by a little vitamin E oil. Wash off the mixture the next morning. Additionally, each day swallow 10 to 15 capsules of liquid garlic in divided dosages (for instance, 3 to 5 at each meal). Pimples and blackheads disappear relatively fast, but severe acne conditions may take as long as six months to clear. For just small patches of acne and pimples, bandage the involved area after applying the combination remedy of vitamin E oil and liquid garlic.

FOR ATHLETE'S FOOT BETWEEN THE TOES: Soak cotton with liquid aged garlic extract and apply to and between the toes affected. Leave the saturated cotton on the toes at night by holding it in place with bed socks. Change the moistened cotton every day. Repeat this treatment as necessary.

FOR COUNTERACTING ALCOHOLIC HANGOVER: Before imbibing alcoholic beverages, take three capsules of liquid aged garlic extract; then, after concluding your alcoholic beverage indulgence, again swallow capsules of aged garlic extract. Use the garlic form that contains vitamin B-1 (thiamine). This should prevent your experiencing any alcoholic hangover.

FOR PREVENTING MOSQUITO ATTACKS: Thirty minutes before hiking in the woods or engaging in other outdoor activity which may be accompanied by mosquito attacks, swallow three capsules of liquid, aged garlic extract contining vitamin B-1.

The renowned herbalist, Dr. John R. Christopher (now deceased), in his book, *School of Natural Healing* (Provo, Utah: BiWorld Publishers, Inc., 1976) lists many medicinal uses for the stinking rose. Among the conditions for which garlic has application are the following: Tuberculosis, asthma, bronchitis, skin diseases, stomach ulcers, leg ulcers, athletes foot, boils, abscesses, epilpsy, worms, high blood pressure, low blood pressure, pimples, carbuncles, tumors, kidney disease, poisonous bites and stings, indigestion, catarrh, pneumonia, earache, infantile convulsions, leprosy, psoriasis, smallpox, intestinal disorders (chronic colitis), respiratory affections and infections, dropsy, body sounds, aging, insect repellant, fevers, nervous and spasmodic coughs, hoarseness, whooping cough, typhus, cholera, hypertension, headaches, backaches, dizziness, vomiting, nausea, diarrhea, dysentery, dyspepsia, heart palpitations, chills, loss of weight, restlessness, diphtheria, colds, colic, pleurisy, intercostal neuralgia, dyspnea, cramps, heartburn, sore throat, rhinitis (clogged and running nose), nicotine poisoning, lip and mouth diseases (ulcers, fissures, etc.), diabetes, ague, pulmonary edema, sciatica, hysteria, ringworm, scrofulous sores, rheumatism, inflamed eyes, eye catarrah, chapped and chafed hands, flatulence, paralysis, neuralgic pains, retention of urine (bladder weakness), heart weakness, eczema, pityriasis, cancers, swollen glands, tubercular joints, and necrosis.

Garlic Goes to the Races

Clarissa McCord of Cloverdale, British Columbia, Canada tells of her use of aged garlic extract in liquid form to combat a virus that attacks horses. Characteristically, the disease passes from horse to horse so as to infect an entire stable. Ms. McCord owns the Cavendish Stables, and she is ever watchful for symptoms of the virus among her horses: fever, coughing, mucus running from nostrils, fatigue, poor feeding, and general disability.

Aged garlic extract was given to the young horses at Cavendish Stables that had contracted this virus. "A bottle of liquid garlic administered on two successive days to each animal does the job of curing," says the horsewoman. "One of my race horses developed the virus symptoms and was to be scratched from the racing program scheduled for the following day. I gave one bottle of liquid garlic to the animal and he improved sufficiently to enter the race. He hit the board first, second, and third.

"In another instance, 'Marty's Winter' and 'Candy Mistico' were given two bottles each of liquid aged garlic extract to control the virus that was running rampant in their bodies. They needed the remedy badly. They went on to race the next day and both finished in the money," McCord assured me. "A two-year old colt named 'Victor' was in such poor shape he was not expected to develop into a race horse. After he took liquid garlic over a brief period, 'Victor' began feeling better and eating lots more. He has now qualified to take part in any races in which he is entered. As a stable owner, I have to admit that taking this aged garlic extract to the races really pays off."

A Veterinarian Detoxifies Dogs and Cats with Liquid Garlic

Gloria Dodd, D.V.M. of Danville, California, has developed a special animal emergency first-aid kit. In the kit Dr. Dodd has included liquid garlic for employment as treatment in animals who come down with virus infections, indigestion, pancreatic and liver problems, and diarrhea. She administers one-quarter teaspoonful of plain aged garlic extract four times a day to the sick animal for two weeks and one-quarter teaspoonful a day thereafter as a prophylactic measure. This procedure, she declares, causes the animals' energy and appetite to increase and makes its coat become glossier. Applying liquid garlic topically each day to the animal's coat also helps to heal skin problems.

One of the most important initial therapies instituted by this veterinarian in her dog and cat patients is a detoxification program. Food is withheld from the animals for 24 hours and they are given enemas to cleanse toxins from the intestines and stomach. Treatment with liquid, aged, garlic concentrate enables poisonous substances to be eliminated naturally. Dr. Dodd says, "With its high concentration of oxygen molecules, the garlic extract has an affinity for attracting the toxins within the animal's stomach and intestines and breaking them down gently and in a non-toxic manner.

"Moreover, the garlic concentrate has been successful in my hands for the treatment of the Parvovirus, a new viral strain found in dogs," she said. "Parvovirus causes severe hemorrhagic gastroenteritis and death. Dogs were dying of acute toxemia and the percentage of mortality was running high in our valley in veterinary practices employing standard orthodox therapies alone. I was able to save every one of my canine patients affected with the Parvovirus.

"Whether they are sick or not," Dr. Dodd added, "I profess the use of aged garlic extract for my patients. Every illness is an accumulation of toxins within the body, be it bacterial, viral, or chemical in origin. These can be prevented with natural methods of detoxification, which includes the daily use of deodorized, aged garlic extract in either tablets, capsules, or liquid. You'll find the product supplied to patients in most wholistic veterinarian practices. The same as they need clean air and clean food, pets and other animals need regular maintenance detoxification."

She concluded, "I believe that what I have said for animals pertains to our own human health as well. I prepare my family's and my own food and make sure that we all take aged garlic extract each day."

For more information, including audiotapes, about Dr. Dodd's therapeutic program for animals using aged garlic extract, contact Gloria Dodd, DVM, Naturo-Vet Service, Inc., 857 El Pintado Road, Danville, California 94526; (415) 847-7759.

In Summary of Garlic's Healing Powers

Garlic has virtues. The herb's healing powers may best be summarized by Sir John Harrington in *The Englishman's Doctor,* published in 1609. Harrington wrote:

Garlic then has power to save
    from death
Bear with it though it maketh
    unsavory breath,
And scorn not garlic like some
    that think
It only maketh men wink and drink
    and stink.

In the modern era, in fact, aged garlic extract is packaged as a deodorized commercial product. It no longer makes you stink; it merely heals what ails you.

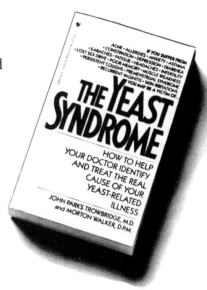